Daily Affirmations for Women

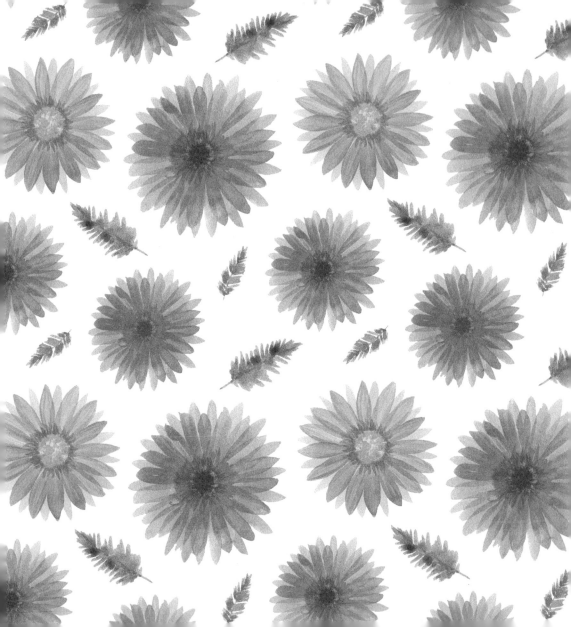

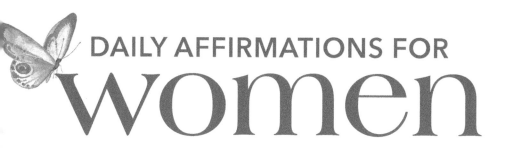

DAILY AFFIRMATIONS FOR
women

Change Your State of Mind with Positive Thinking

Christine Rose Elle

**ROCKRIDGE
PRESS**

For general information on our other products and services or to obtain technical support, please contact our Customer Care Department within the United States at (866) 744-2665, or outside the United States at (510) 253-0500.

Rockridge Press publishes its books in a variety of electronic and print formats. Some content that appears in print may not be available in electronic books, and vice versa.

Interior and Cover Designer: Jenny Paredes
Art Producer: Maya Melenchuk
Editor: Olivia Bartz
Production Editor: Jax Berman
Production Manager: Eric Pier-Hocking

All images used under license from Shutterstock
Author photo courtesy of Harper Point Photography, Ventura CA

Paperback ISBN: 978-1-63807-976-7
eBook ISBN: 978-1-63807-660-5
R0

To all the courageous women who enter the arena of self-discovery. May your bravery inspire generations to come.

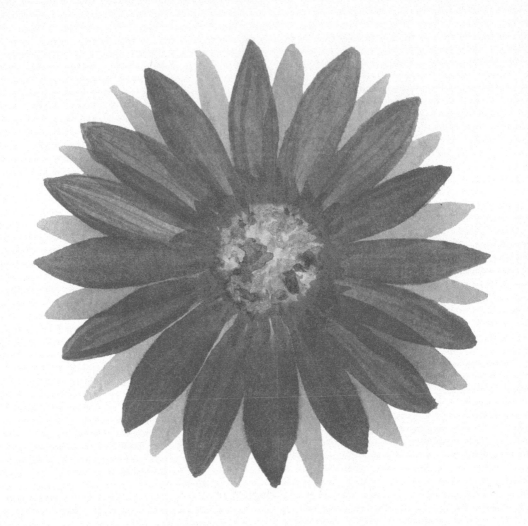

CONTENTS

INTRODUCTION

D id you know you have a superpower in your pocket? It's the power of positive thinking!

But positive thinking isn't about false optimism or blowing off how you truly feel. It's about learning to think positively to face challenges in a skillful way that fosters emotional empowerment.

And it gets even better. Engaging with positivity this way also gives you more confidence and enhances your wellbeing. I discovered this through my own personal wellness journey, while working with women in my coaching practice who were struggling to process difficult emotions in a healthy and transformative way.

I first encountered affirmations years ago while reading about the power of positive thinking as a way to overcome my habit of negative self-talk. Affirmations are written or verbal reminders of the psychological strengths you possess within yourself. Using them helps you create a strong foundation of emotional support, especially when combined with insightful actions like the exercises in this book. Affirmations work by helping you internalize the words and phrases to transform them into positive personal beliefs.

Here's the deal when it comes to developing your positivity: human brains are hardwired to highlight the negative. It takes five positive interactions to balance one negative one—that's quite the bias! If it goes unchecked, negativity can consume the best parts of yourself. Using positive affirmations will help you lay a foundation to manage your emotions with love and support.

Notice I didn't say that by using affirmations, you won't ever have difficult thoughts or feelings, because you will. But using affirmations to practice positive thinking gives you the skills to manage your emotions in a meaningful way and can even affect self-care and confidence.

You can interpret and implement the affirmations in this book in any way that feels right. Alongside them are Positively You sections that offer strategies to develop a more positive outlook on life. Each page will support you with what you need in the moment, whether it's a simple positive reminder for starting your day or a pick-me-up after a stressful experience.

Your relationship to positive thinking is unique, and it's yours to craft and design, but it's not a device for shutting off difficult emotions. It's a process for stimulating profound insights that support a long-term perspective of positivity with tools you can pull out of your pocket anytime, anywhere. (See what I mean? Superpower!)

HOW TO MAKE AFFIRMATIONS PART OF YOUR DAILY LIFE

If you are someone who has tried affirmations only to have your initial excitement fade, here are some practical ideas for engaging with affirmations so they become part of your daily routine:

Use them as journaling prompts. If you have a daily journaling routine or want to start one, write an affirmation at the top of the page and jot down what comes to mind. Don't overthink it. Five minutes of stream-of-consciousness writing is enough to create a positive effect.

Work them into meditation practice. You don't have to be a seasoned meditator to enjoy the benefits of gentle breathing and focused thought. Pick an affirmation that resonates with you and hold it in your mind's eye. Breathe into it and let it be there.

Post them in your favorite places. Write your favorite affirmations down on sticky notes and leave them in places you frequent daily. Place them on your mirror, by the sink, or near the door where you hang your keys. Change them often. You can get used to seeing things a certain way, so changing the location or message will have a bigger impact.

Read them before bed. Drift off with your affirmation in mind and let your subconscious do the work.

Text them to a friend. Sharing daily affirmations with people you love is a great way to support yourself and express compassion.

Schedule them into your phone's notifications. This is especially helpful when you know you're going to have a challenging or busy day.

Create a mood board that features your favorite affirmations. Bonus points if you collect inspiring visuals with websites like Pinterest to support what the affirmation means to you.

Working with affirmations is inspiring and fun and doesn't require a lot of time. If using them starts to feel like work, that's your cue to get creative with arts and crafts or use a pocket journal. Allow them to become part of your daily wellness and self-care routine by making them approachable and easy.

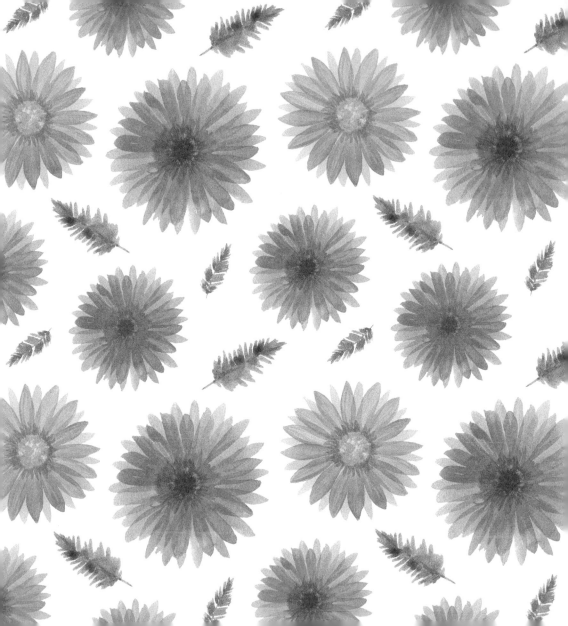

Positively

You &

Affirmations

Positively You:
Relationships

Meaningful relationships make life beautiful, but sometimes they can be challenging. Observing how you connect and engage with other people can tell you a lot about yourself and what you need from relationships, whether it's more intimacy, compassion, or forgiveness. Do you feel closer to others when you engage one-on-one, or do you feel energized by mingling in small groups? This might sound a little clichéd, but it's too important not to mention: having a loving relationship with *yourself* is essential for substantial, healthy connections with others. If you're feeling disjointed in your relationships, take time to reconnect with your needs. Knowing yourself and sharing the best parts of who you are helps cultivate intimacy and healthier relationships.

I cultivate intimacy and connection
by sharing the beautiful and
imperfect parts of myself.

I seek experiences that allow me to connect deeply with others.

I inspire people when I share
my dreams and goals.

I accept and love myself unconditionally so I can do the same for the ones I love.

I nurture relationships that are
loving and supportive, and I welcome
love and support in return.

My sense of empathy helps me
make friends and sustain
loving relationships.

Positively You:
Strengths

Have you ever wondered why some activities or projects are fun and enjoyable, while others aren't as much? When you experience satisfaction and pleasure in what you do, it's likely that you're engaging your natural strengths. Your strengths are qualities like courage, love of learning, and humor that create a positive state of mind when you apply them.

There are several different ways to determine your strengths:

- Take an online quiz.
- Write an inventory of your past achievements and think about what connects them to one another.
- Make a list of your interests and highlight what they have in common.

By identifying your strengths and engaging them in your next project, you might experience a boost to your sense of positivity. Want even more life fulfillment? Find a way to share your strengths with others.

I use my strengths to tackle
challenging situations.

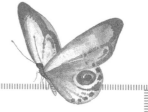

I am worthy of dedicating time
to build my personal strengths.

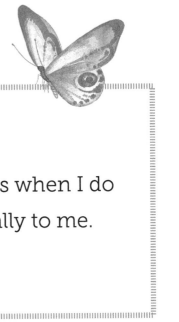

I delight in the possibilities when I do things that come naturally to me.

I'm dedicated to nurturing
my sources of inner strength.

I'm energized by trying new
things and cultivating them into
things I love.

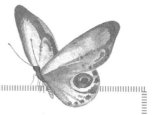

I'm building lifelong fulfillment by sharing with others what I do best.

Positively You:
Inner Wisdom

Y ou are wiser than you know. That's because you've earned inner wisdom along every step of your unique journey through life. There are different types of inner wisdom based on intellectual, emotional, and intuitive mindsets.

Here's a brief breakdown:

- Your intellectual mind is useful when you are problem-solving or making tough decisions.

- Your emotional mind is useful when you are reaching for compassion or forgiveness.

- Your intuitive mind is the blend and balance of your ideas, thoughts, and emotions and is useful for navigating everything.

When personal trust and inner wisdom act together, blending both ideas and emotions, you'll experience more positive outcomes in challenging situations. Trust that your inner wisdom has your back.

When I'm uncertain or in conflict,
I trust myself to make the
right decisions.

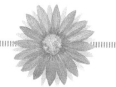

My negative thoughts are an
invitation to get curious about
my feelings.

I am worthy and wise.

I celebrate unique experiences
that enrich my inner wisdom.

I allow myself to keenly listen to my thoughts and feel my emotions.

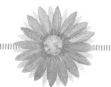

My deep sources of inner wisdom
guide me through life
with confidence.

I quiet my mind and connect to
the depths of my deepest self.

Positively You:
Gratitude Practice

P racticing gratitude is known to boost your overall sense of happiness and wellbeing. A simple and powerful way to do this is to keep a journal. Gratitude journaling is a tried-and-true activity that creates massive transformation. To keep this habit fresh, routinely list things that give you a sense of delight. When you capture these little wonders on paper, your sense of appreciation for the good things will amplify. If you find yourself overthinking it, losing interest after a few days, or seeing gratitude journaling as just another chore, don't worry. The best way to overcome this is to keep things super simple. Here's how:

- Get a small notebook that's only for gratitude reflection. List three items of delight or thanks per day.

- List three people who help, support, or inspire you per day.

- Do it at the same time each day.

That's it!

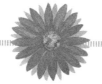

My eyes are open to my
many blessings.

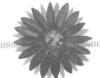

I feel peaceful and whole
when I focus on gratitude.

My gratitude toward others fills
me with positivity
and possibility.

I choose mindfulness and gratitude to help me enter the present moment.

I appreciate the wonder of
everyday magic in small things.

I give my dreams and goals vitality by
practicing gratitude for the support
I receive.

I'm grateful for the challenging life lessons I experience because they allow me to improve self-love.

Positively You:
Flow

A wonderful source of positivity and happiness comes from the ability to access your state of flow. What exactly is flow? It's the mental state that emerges from being fully engaged in a task or activity. The task might feel challenging, but it isn't overwhelming or frustrating. You have the sense that time is standing still. The ability to access the state of flow on a regular basis, especially while doing something enjoyable, is a dynamic form of happiness and life satisfaction. To find flow and improve your sense of wellbeing, practice activities that require focus and a balance between effort and skill. What are the activities in which you find your sense of flow? Painting, writing, or playing a sport are great examples.

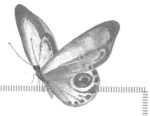

I have what it takes to focus
on things that matter to me.

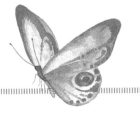

I can show up and be imperfect
doing what I love.

I find the balance between effort and
skill when I'm in a flow state.

Making mistakes is part
of developing my best self.

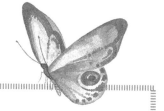

I learn about myself when I step
outside my comfort zone.

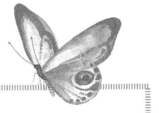

Meaningful things are worthy
of my full attention.

Nurturing my flow experiences
allows me to live more fully.

Positively You:
Savoring

Tap into the power of savoring by paying attention to something with conscious appreciation. This can be done with moments from the past, present, and future. To savor a present moment, tune in to the sights, sounds, textures, and smells around you. To savor a moment from the past, allow memories and emotions to wash over you and revel in them. What was significant about that experience? To savor a future moment, think about the anticipation you might feel and the hopes associated with it.

Savoring is different from meditation or daydreaming. It's about embracing an experience wholeheartedly and allowing emotions to arrive from your senses and wash over you.

I use my senses to savor meaningful experiences.

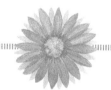

I purposefully and mindfully
give my attention to experiences
that enrich my life.

By consciously savoring wonderful
moments, I am enhancing my wellbeing.

I visualize things to come with positivity, wonder, and appreciation.

My cherished memories
bring me joy in the present.

I allow myself to simply breathe
and embrace the
current moment.

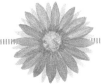

I nourish my inner child by giving myself permission to reconnect with playful memories.

Positively You:
Pleasure, Passion, Purpose

Happiness and positivity often stroll hand-in-hand. Did you know there are several types of happiness? The three categories of happiness are pleasure, passion, and purpose.

Pleasure is short-term happiness from things like eating a delicious meal or getting a promotion. **Passion**-related happiness emerges from activities that allow you to be significantly engaged while using your strengths, also known as flow.

Purpose-related happiness comes from using your strengths for the benefit of others.

Life satisfaction and fulfillment happen when passion- and purpose-driven happiness come together. Perhaps you have a creative business that supports dog rescues, or you develop courses that teach people how to make art. When you merge your passion and purpose, pleasure is like the whipped cream and cherry on top. How do you experience engaging, meaningful forms of happiness?

My passion and purpose
converge when I'm
engaged in what I do.

I choose happiness when
the activities I do
are meaningful.

I'm worthy of living a life that
is pleasurable, passionate,
and purposeful.

Today I am open to happiness
in all its forms.

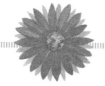

My life is filled with connection
to others and positivity
from helping others.

I deserve and enjoy short-term
pleasures, but I also embrace
the effort needed for
long-term happiness.

Positively You:
Permission

Are you holding yourself back from something you really want because you need permission? There are two ways to recognize if you need to give yourself permission. You may desire something that seems indulgent or decadent but really isn't, such as taking a nap or investing in a fun course. Or perhaps you recognize your desire is attached to an outdated belief (maybe something you learned as a kid) or it's in conflict with someone else's belief.

Here are a few ways to give yourself permission:

◆ Accept and acknowledge your desires and the feelings that come along with them.

◆ Be willing to make mistakes.

◆ Be flexible with people who might not understand your choices.

◆ Embrace the unknown.

By giving yourself permission to explore your curiosities and interests, you'll build the positive and joyful life you deserve.

I give myself permission to invest
in my health, wellbeing,
and self-actualization.

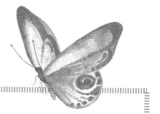

I am allowed to take care of myself
and meet my needs.

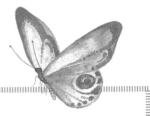

When I validate my own emotions,

I give myself permission to feel.

The permission I give myself today is a necessary part of my self-discovery.

With love and compassion,
I allow myself to be imperfect.

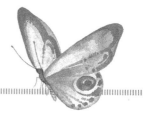

When I step out of my own way,
I give myself permission to
develop and prosper.

Positively You:
Boundaries

Boundaries are expressions of feelings, beliefs, or needs that support your sense of fairness, self-worth, and emotional wellbeing. How do you know if you need a boundary? There is one telltale feeling that signals the need for a boundary: resentment. Resentment is triggered when you feel like someone isn't respecting your time, energy, or needs.

Communicating a boundary is the first step to resolving resentment. Types of boundaries include but aren't limited to: personal, professional, physical, emotional, time-oriented, sexual, and financial. Clarifying a boundary has three components: describing the triggering event, the consequence of the event, and stating the desire or need. Making your boundary known might go something like this: "When you make plans without checking in with me [triggering event], it makes me feel unheard [consequence]. Please check my calendar or text me so I can be included [need]."

Boundary established! It takes a little practice, but setting boundaries is positive and healthy for everyone.

I communicate my needs without
shame or personal judgment.

Looking after my boundaries is nonnegotiable for my wellbeing and self-worth.

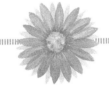

I'm in charge of identifying, communicating, and speaking my needs and limits.

I am worthy of being
heard and respected.

I'm allowed to say no to things that aren't a good fit for me, and yes to the things that are.

My boundaries support my commitment to personal growth, self-care, and health.

Positively You:
Flourishing

Flourishing is a state of wellbeing in which you're vividly in touch with your potential. There are different ways you can experience flourishing:

- **Emotional flourishing:** When you experience more positive than negative feelings and you are skillful with managing your emotions.

- **Relational flourishing:** When you have positive exchanges with loving people in your life.

- **Purposeful flourishing:** When you have a clear sense of what you value and want to accomplish in life.

- **Accomplished flourishing:** When you are using your strengths and talents to set and achieve goals.

These are the building blocks for flourishing with positivity and purpose. They fluctuate and change, so be sure to check in from time to time to see which areas need nurturing.

Today, I'm planting the seeds that
will help me grow and
flourish tomorrow.

I flourish by skillfully managing
and feeling my emotions.

True healing emerges when I listen
to the unsettled parts of myself.

Today is filled with possibility, and I'm empowered to set my own pace.

I make decisions that allow me
to flourish and thrive.

I surround myself with
positive, loving people who
support my flourishing.

Positively You:
Self-Empathy

"Be nice to yourself." It's a familiar expression in self-help for good reason. When you treat yourself with empathy in self-talk and behavior, you strengthen all the same positive emotions and feelings of connection that you experience in your most nurturing relationships. The amount of kindness you show yourself will change the way you feel about yourself.

One way to practice self-empathy and really bolster those feelings of positivity is by practicing mindfulness. For example, in loving-kindness meditation, you are invited to send love to yourself and others by speaking and repeating mantras. These mantras include sentiments for the people you cherish and the people you find difficult. Mantras include things like "May I be happy and peaceful," or "May they be liberated from suffering." Intentionally using mantras boosts empathy toward yourself and others, so it's a win/win!

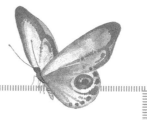

I accept who I am and
give myself permission
to love all of me.

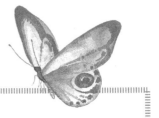

I am worthy of the same
love I give to others.

The more empathy I have toward myself, the more I have to share.

Self-empathy empowers me
to take bold actions
that support my wellbeing.

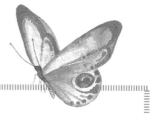

I am grateful for my kind nature
and the love I supply myself.

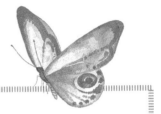

Even when I misstep, I support myself with love and kindness.

Positively You:
Optimism

When you hear the word *optimism*, does it trigger feelings of how you should feel, but often don't? Sometimes being optimistic can seem impossible because it's incongruent with your current mood. Optimism is simply feeling hopeful about future outcomes. Your mood is independent from the things you are hopeful for, so don't worry if you're not oozing sunshine and rainbows. You can live optimistically by identifying expectations attached to a situation and acknowledging the outcome you desire.

Ask yourself: are you filtering things through a negative lens? Negativity can be an old habit that needs your awareness. Living optimistically means being committed to living vibrantly and relishing the challenges life throws your way, the wins as well as the stumbles. When you embrace positivity and optimism, you're saying "yes" to excitement and hope.

My optimistic nature
flows freely through me.

I allow my range of feelings
to emerge. I accept them
and choose to be optimistic.

Good things happen when I acknowledge my hopes and expectations. Great things happen when I'm open and optimistic about the outcome.

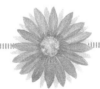

Each new day, my optimism fills
me with gratitude, hope, and possibility.

I let go of negativity through
my ability to hope for good things.

My future is enriched by the
positive opportunities
I make the most of today.

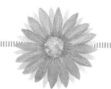

Positively You:
Forgiveness

Forgiveness means letting go of the negative emotions and beliefs that come from a charged experience. Instead of letting those feelings consume you, forgiveness lets you focus on what truly makes you happy. Getting to a place of acceptance around painful events is an emotional journey. Forgiving someone is an odyssey that will challenge your spirit and ultimately set you free, but not all forgiveness is equal. It's easier to excuse your roommate for eating your leftovers than it is to forgive your ex for cheating on you and draining your bank account.

But the most important thing to remember is that forgiving isn't for *them*. It's for *you*.

You have to be willing to go through bad experiences and feel the feelings, including sadness, guilt, rage, and all the other emotions you typically avoid. That's the hard part. Allowing yourself to process what you feel through journaling or inviting your emotions to tea will bring you closer to letting go. You'll feel light, inspired, and whole. That's the positively lovely part.

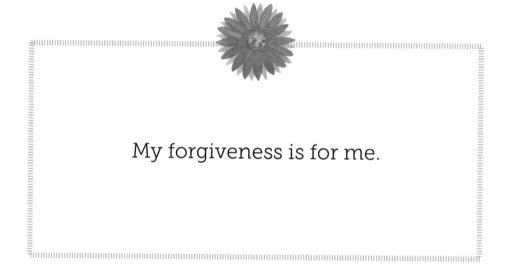

My forgiveness is for me.

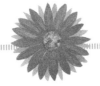

I release the hold that resentment

and anger have on me.

I am free.

I choose to let go of the hurt.

I uplift myself by forgiving.

I forgive myself for past mistakes
and trade shame for self-love.

My life is filled with peace

as I learn to forgive.

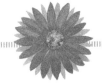

I find tranquility by being gentle
with myself and accepting what
I can't change.

Positively You:
Clarified Values

Did you know you can nurture positivity and purpose by clarifying your values? Let's refresh for a moment. Your values are like a personal filter for life. Defining them is essential for wellbeing because it helps you integrate them into what you do. If you know your values include creativity, curiosity, and grit, you're able to use them as a filter for how you spend your time, energy, and money. Take time to think about what is truly meaningful to you and how you like to live your life. Ultimately, clarifying your values will bring more positive engagement and joy to the things you do and how you do them. If you've previously taken time to define your values, consider revisiting and updating them, because they usually change over time.

I am outgrowing old beliefs that keep me stuck and am connecting to the values that make me strong.

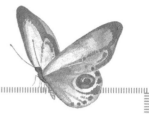

My values guide me to a deeper
awareness of my life's desires.

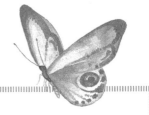

I spend my time, energy, and resources in alignment with my most cherished beliefs.

I focus on the things that
create positive change.

I'm in control of defining the values
that are meaningful to me.

Positively You:
Authenticity

How do you know if you are living authentically? While it's something that gets talked about a lot, it's easy to misunderstand what it means to be authentic. Authenticity is something you can intuitively know when observing it in someone else. Likewise, you deeply feel it when someone isn't authentic. But what exactly is it?

Authenticity is simply behaving in ways that align with your true feelings and personal beliefs. The path to discovering your authentic self goes something like this:

- Seek to understand who you are: your thoughts, beliefs, and values.

- Behave in ways that align with those beliefs.

- Share your authentic qualities with other people.

- Accept and love yourself.

Nurturing your authenticity is part self-discovery journey, part inspired action. Living authentically allows you to speak your truth and become the most spirited, positive version of yourself.

I support myself in acknowledging
my true feelings.

My beliefs are in alignment
with my actions.

I deserve to live authentically.

I'm allowed to speak my truth.

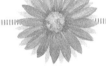

I love and accept all aspects
of who I am, even the parts
that are difficult.

My authentic self emerges because of my curiosity and commitment to self-discovery.

I am blessed to share the
best parts of myself with
the people I love.

Positively You:
Seeking Beauty

I f you've been taught that appreciation of beauty is superficial, it's time to do a conscious uncoupling of that idea. Here's why. When you experience and appreciate beauty in the world, it stimulates feelings of transcendence and wonder. You forget about your small self and relate to the world in a hallowed and humbled way. The stars sparkle and your heart opens wide. It's a powerful thing to stand in awe of beauty.

Recognizing the sublime also inspires lifelong creativity. How did you feel the last time you watched a brilliant sunset or waves lapping on a beach? Maybe you felt otherworldly wholeness while observing a work of art or listening to your favorite playlist. Discover and appreciate what you find beautiful. It's a vibrant part of living and building a life of positivity and gratitude.

I cultivate experiences that guide me
to beautiful moments.

I honor my inner beauty and
let it shine out to the world.

I take time to observe and recognize life's beauty.

My life is enriched by sharing
beautiful experiences with others.

I celebrate special events in life by noticing the beauty, artistry, and effort that went into creating them.

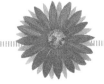

Appreciation of beauty allows
me to experience things that are
bigger than myself.

Positively You:
Inner Peace

Developing inner peace has a lot to do with practicing acceptance. That doesn't mean approving of things you don't agree with or consenting to things you don't want to do. It only means that you acknowledge what "is" and are aware of any resistance you have to that reality. Sometimes things beyond your control are hard to accept, especially when they are truly unfair. But there are ways to quiet your internal conflict depending on the level of disturbance to your inner peace.

When you feel unsettled, nurture yourself with what soothes you: nature walks, bubble baths, gentle exercise, meditation, or whatever works for you. Be gentle. To regain your inner balance, accept your emotions and acknowledge what you can't control. Nourish your inner calm and remain in the present moment to greet the peace that lives here.

I take care of myself by listening
to my needs and protecting my
inner peace.

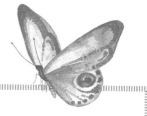

I decide how much access emotionally turbulent people have to me.

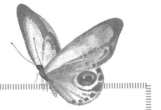

Cultivating inner peace is a priority.

Embracing peace allows me
to hear the calm within.

I see chaotic moments as an opportunity to practice self-care.

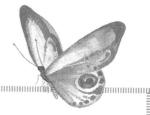

I no longer resist reality
to avoid the emotions
that I'm afraid to feel.

Positively You:
Your Calling

People who have identified their calling in life are generally happier and more positive. Everyone has a calling: a purposeful way to use your skills and strengths that leads to fulfillment. Sometimes your calling and career are the same, but not always. The big difference is that your calling is something that gives you a sense of positivity and meaning. Your career is a path that pays the bills and leads to opportunities and progress, but it doesn't always lead to happiness. The hardest part about finding your calling can be identifying how all your interests and passions fit together. The best way to nail it down is to experiment and see what sparks. Take time to identify the positive aspects of what you try and how they make you feel. If your calling isn't clear, just keep going—it emerges as you do.

I am blessed to have a calling that
emerges more each day.

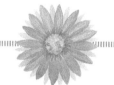

I listen to my intuition
and trust my choices.

I'm brave enough to embrace
challenges that support my goals
and interests.

I easily find inspiration that fuels my curiosity and ignites my potential.

Everything I do takes me a step closer
to my calling in life.

I'm committed to self-discovery.

My curiosity nurtures my calling.

Positively You:
Believe in Yourself

Confidence, trusting your capabilities, and sharing your truth all add up to believing in yourself. Confidence is about showing up, doing the thing, and being ready to accept the outcome knowing you tried your best. It means knowing you can rely on yourself to stand up and take care of your needs. In order to share your truth, you must be willing to experience discomfort for something you believe in.

If you need a confidence boost to better believe in yourself, here are some things to try:

- Set some new goals. Remember to make them clear and time-specific.

- Make an inventory of your accomplishments—you've done so much more than you think.

- Don't forget to engage your strengths.

- Define what success is for you.

Believing in yourself is simply taking time to acknowledge how far you've come, and knowing deep down that you have the courage to keep going.

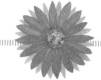

I have everything I need within myself to show up and be my best.

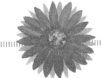

When it doesn't serve me, I let it go.

I check in with my needs
to mindfully go at my own pace.

I use my strengths to navigate
new opportunities.

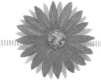

I trust my inner wisdom
to make confident choices.

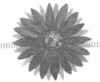

Good things happen when
I define my self-worth.

I'm in control of what
I allow in my life.

References

Csikszentmihalyi, Mihaly. *Flow: The Psychology of Optimal Experience*. New York: Harper Perennial, 1990.

Jankowski, P. J., Steven J. Sandage, Chance A. Bell, Don E. Davis, Emma Porter, Mackenzie Jessen, Christine L. Motzny, Kaitlin V. Ross, and Jesse Owen. "Virtue, Flourishing, and Positive Psychology in Psychotherapy: An Overview and Research Prospectus." *Psychotherapy* 57, no. 3 (September 2020): 291–309. doi.org/10.1037/pst0000285.

Linehan, Marsha M. *Building a Life Worth Living: A Memoir*. New York: Random House, 2020.

Lyubomirsky, Sonja. *The How of Happiness: A Practical Guide to Getting the Life You Want*. New York: Piatkus, 2010.

Moore, Catherine. "What Is the Negativity Bias and How Can It Be Overcome?" PositivePsychology.com. April 26, 2021. PositivePsychology. com/3-steps-negativity-bias.

Ramirez, Daniela. "Savoring in Psychology: 21 Exercises and Interventions to Appreciate Life." PositivePsychology.com. September 10, 2021. PositivePsychology.com/savoring.

Seligman, Martin E. P. *Authentic Happiness: Using the New Positive Psychology to Realize Your Potential for Lasting Fulfillment*. New York: Free Press, 2002.

Acknowledgements

Thank *you* for investing in your one, precious life! Thanks to Morgan for all the love and support. Thanks to Crystal Nero, Kim Caruthers, and the amazing team at Callisto. Gratitude to my friends who have shared my work and encouraged me with kind words. Blessings to my celestial angel, Julie Weller, whose last words to me are etched on my heart: "Never stop sharing your beauty with the world."
    I never ever will.

About the Author

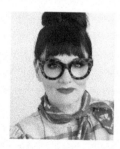 **Christine Rose Elle** is the author of *The Happy Empath: A Survival Guide for Highly Sensitive People* and *52-Week Inspirational Journal: Find Your Spark.* Her work has been featured in publications worldwide. She inspires people to find emotional freedom and develop their creativity through online courses, journaling techniques, and coaching.